Keto Diet Cookbook

A Complete Ketogenic Cookbook To Enjoy Your Meals for Beginners, from Breakfast to Dessert

Amanda Brooks

Table of Content

SMOOTHIES & BREAKFAST

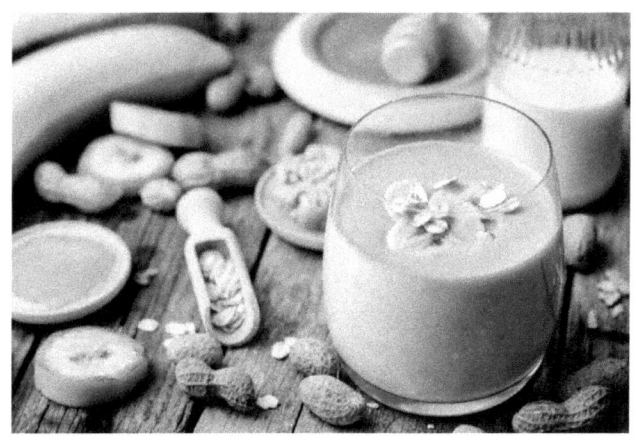

Apple Ginger Blueberry Smoothie

Preparation Time: 5 minutes Cooking Time: 5 minutes Serve: 2

Ingredients:

- 1/2 apple
- 1 tsp MCT oil
- 1/2 tbsp collagen powder
- 1 tsp ginger
- 1 cup unsweetened coconut milk
- 1/2 cup coconut yogurt
- 15 blueberries

Directions:

1. Add all ingredients into the blender and blend until smooth.
2. Serve and enjoy.

Nutritional Value (Amount per Serving):

Calories 169

Fat 15 g

Carbohydrates 5 g

Sugar 2 g

Protein 4 g

Cholesterol 5 mg

Choco Sunflower Butter Smoothie

Preparation Time: 5 minutes Cooking Time: 5 minutes Serve: 1

Ingredients:

- 1/3 cup unsweetened coconut milk
- 1/4 cup ice
- 1/2 tsp vanilla
- 1 tsp unsweetened cocoa powder
- 2/3 cup water
- 2 tbsp sunflower seed butter

Directions:

- Add all ingredients into the blender and blend until smooth.
- Serve and enjoy.

Nutritional Value (Amount per Serving):

Calories 379

Fat 34.6 g

Carbohydrates 13 g

Sugar 3 g

Protein 8.5 g

Cholesterol 0 mg

PORK, BEEF &
LAMB RECIPES

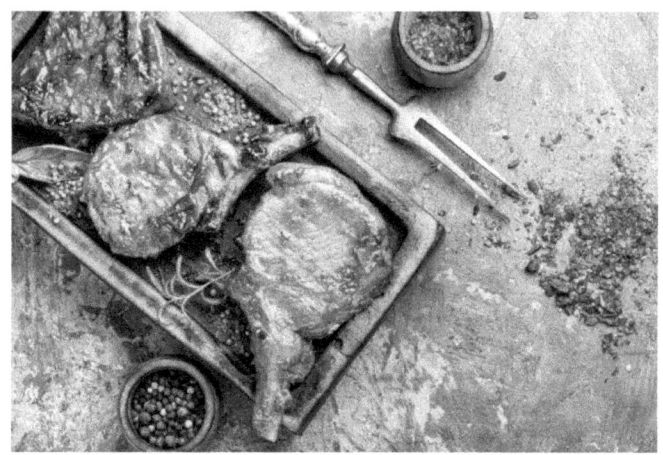

Pan Fry Pork Chops

Preparation Time: 10 minutes Cooking Time: 8

minutes

Serve: 4

Ingredients:

- 4 pork chops, boneless
- 2 tbsp olive oil
- 1/4 tsp onion powder
- 1/4 tsp garlic powder
- 1/4 tsp pepper
- Salt

Directions:

Heat oil in cast iron skillet over high heat.

1. Season pork chops with garlic powder, onion powder, pepper, and salt.
2. Sear pork chops in hot oil about 3-4 minutes on each side.
3. Serve and enjoy.

Nutritional Value (Amount per Serving):

Calories 317

Fat 26 g

Carbohydrates 0.3 g

Sugar 0.1 g

Protein 18 g

Cholesterol 69 mg

SEAFOOD & FISH RECIPES

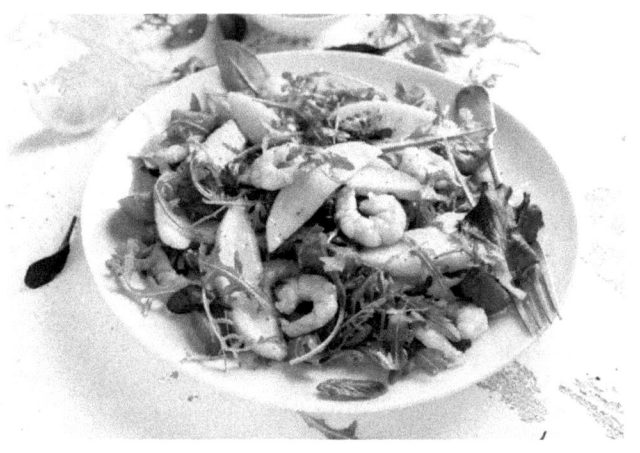

Spinach Shrimp Alfredo

Preparation Time: 10 minutes Cooking Time: 15
minutes

Serve: 2

Ingredients:

- 1/2 lb shrimp, deveined
- 2 garlic cloves, minced
- 2 tbsp onion, chopped
- 1 cup fresh spinach, chopped
- 1/2 cup heavy cream
- 1 tbsp butter
- Pepper
- Salt

Directions:

1. Melt butter in a pan over medium heat.
2. Add onion, garlic and shrimp in the pan and sauté for 3 minutes.
3. Add remaining ingredients and simmer for 7 minutes or until cooked.
4. Serve and enjoy.

Nutritional Value (Amount per Serving):

Calories 300

Fat 19 g

Carbohydrates 5 g

Sugar 0.5 g

Protein 27 g

Cholesterol 295 mg

Avocado Shrimp Salad

Preparation Time: 10 minutes Cooking Time: 10 minutes

Serve: 6

Ingredients:

- 1 lb shrimp
- 3 bacon slices, cooked and crumbled
- 1/4 cup feta cheese, crumbled
- 1 tbsp lemon juice
- 1/2 cup tomatoes, chopped
- 2 avocados, chopped
- 2 garlic cloves, minced
- 1 tbsp olive oil
- Pepper
- Salt

Directions:

1. Heat oil in a pan over medium heat.
2. Add garlic and sauté for minute.
3. Add shrimp, pepper, and salt and cook for 5-7 minutes. Remove from heat and set aside.
4. Meanwhile, add remaining ingredients to the large mixing bowl.

5. Add shrimp and toss well.

6. Cover and place in fridge for 1 hour.

7. Serve and enjoy.

Nutritional Value (Amount per Serving):

Calories 268

Fat 18 g

Carbohydrates 8.1 g

Sugar 1.1 g

Protein 19.6 g

Cholesterol 165 mg

MEATLESS
MEALS

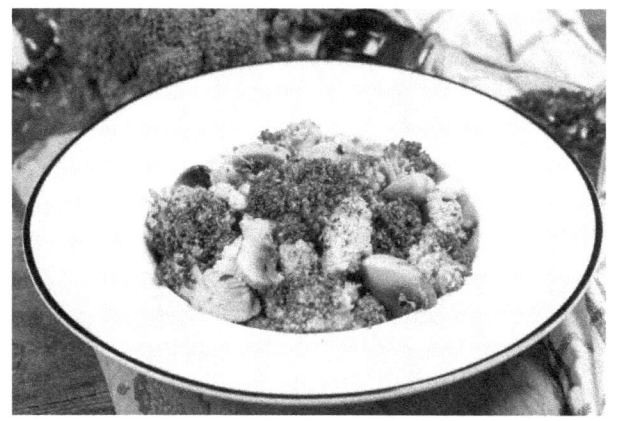

Cauliflower Broccoli Rice

Preparation Time: 10 minutes Cooking Time: 8
minutes Serve: 4

Ingredients:

- 1 cup broccoli, process into rice
- 3 cups cauliflower rice
- 1/4 cup mascarpone cheese
- 1/2 cup parmesan cheese, shredded
- 1/8 tsp ground cinnamon
- ¼ tsp garlic powder
- ¼ tsp onion powder
- 1/4 tsp pepper
- 1 tbsp butter, melted
- 1/2 tsp salt

Directions:

1. In a heat-safe bowl, mix together cauliflower, nutmeg, garlic powder, onion powder, butter, broccoli, pepper, and salt and microwave for 4 minutes.
2. Stir well and microwave for 2 minutes more.
3. Add cheese and microwave for 2 minutes.
4. Add mascarpone cheese and stir until it looks creamy.
5. Serve and enjoy.

Nutritional Value (Amount per Serving):

Calories 135

Fat 10 g

Carbohydrates 6 g

Sugar 2 g

Protein 8 g

Cholesterol 30 mg

SOUPS, STEWS & SALADS

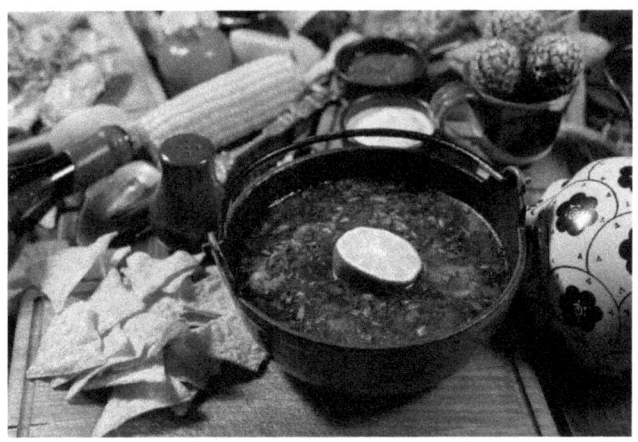

Hearty Cabbage Beef Soup

Preparation Time: 10 minutes Cooking Time: 45 minutes
Serve: 10

Ingredients:

- 2 lbs ground beef

- 4 cups chicken stock

- 10 oz Rotel tomatoes, diced

- 3 cube bouillon

- 1 large cabbage head, chopped

- ½ tsp cumin powder

- 2 garlic cloves, minced
- ¼ onion, diced
- Pepper
- Salt

Directions:

1. Brown the meat in pan over medium heat.
2. Add onion and cook until soften.
3. Transfer meat mixture to the stock pot.
4. Add remaining ingredients to the stock pot stir well and bring to boil over high heat.
5. Turn heat to medium-low and simmer for 45 minutes.

Nutritional Value (Amount per Serving):

Calories 260

Fat 18 g

Carbohydrates 5 g

Sugar 2 g

Protein 15 g

Cholesterol 64 mg

Veggie Shrimp Soup

Preparation Time: 10 minutes Cooking Time: 5
hours

Serve: 6

Ingredients:

- oz shrimp
- 4 cups chicken broth
- 2 cups heavy cream
- 4 oz turnip, diced
- 5 oz broccoli florets
- 6 oz cauliflower florets
- 4 cups water
- 2 bouillon cubes

Directions:

1. Add all ingredients except shrimp into the slow cooker and stir well.
2. Cover and cook on low for 4 hours 30 minutes.
3. Add shrimp and stir well. Cover and cook for 30 minutes more.
4. Season with salt and serve.

Nutritional Value (Amount per Serving):

Calories 345

Fat 31 g

Carbohydrates 6 g

Sugar 1 g

Protein 10 g

Cholesterol 205 mg

BRUNCH & DINNER

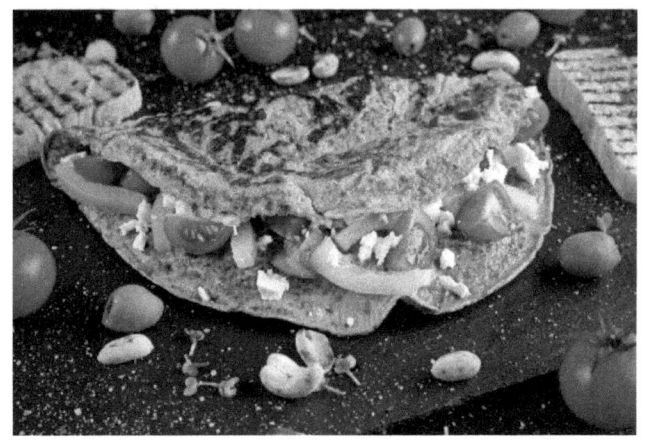

Cheese Almond Pancakes

Preparation Time: 10 minutes Cooking Time: 10 minutes

Serve: 4

Ingredients:

- 4 eggs
- 1/4 tsp cinnamon
- 1/2 cup cream cheese
- 1/2 cup almond flour
- 1 tbsp butter, melted

Directions:

1. Add all ingredients into the blender and blend until combined.
2. Melt butter in a pan over medium heat.
3. Pour 3 tablespoons of batter per pancake and cook for 2 minutes on each side.
4. Serve and enjoy.

Nutritional Value (Amount per Serving):

Calories 271

Fat 25 g

Carbohydrates 5 g

Sugar 1 g

Protein 10.8 g

Cholesterol 203 mg

DESSERTS & DRINKS

Cheesecake Fat Bombs

Preparation Time: 10 minutes Cooking Time: 10 minutes

Serve: 24

Ingredients:

- 8 oz cream cheese
- 1 ½ tsp vanilla
- 2 tbsp erythritol
- 4 oz coconut oil
- 4 oz heavy cream

Directions:

1. Add all ingredients into the mixing bowl and beat using immersion blender until creamy.
2. Pour batter into the mini cupcake liner and place in refrigerator until set.
3. Serve and enjoy.

Nutritional Value (Amount per Serving):

Calories 90

Fat 9.8 g

Carbohydrates 1.4 g

Sugar 0.1 g

Protein 0.8 g

Cholesterol 17 mg

BREAKFAST RECIPES

Keto Iced Matcha Latte

Serves: 1

Prep Time: 10 mins Ingredients

Total Carbohydrate 1.5g 1% Dietary Fiber 0.4g 1%
Total Sugars 0.9g Protein 0.5g

- 1 teaspoon matcha powder, high quality

- 1 cup water

  - ½ tablespoon coconut oil

  - ½ teaspoon Stevia powder

  - 1 cup organic coconut milk, frozen into ice cubes

Directions

1. Put all the ingredients except collagen powder in a high powered blender.
2. Pulse until completely smooth and pour into a glass to serve.

Nutrition Amount per serving

Calories 175

Total Fat 17.8g 23% Saturated Fat 16.9g 84% Cholesterol 0mg 0%

Sodium 10mg 0%

Total Carbohydrate 1g 0% Dietary Fiber 2g 7%

Cauliflower Toast with Avocado

Serves: 2

Prep Time: 20 mins

Ingredients

- 1 large egg
- 1 small head cauliflower, grated
- 1 medium avocado, pitted and chopped
- ¾ cup mozzarella cheese, shredded
- Salt and black pepper, to taste

Directions

1. Preheat the oven to 420°F and line a baking sheet with parchment.
2. Place the cauliflower in a microwave safe bowl and microwave for about 7 minutes on high.
3. Spread on paper towels to drain after the cauliflower has completely cooled and press with a clean towel to remove excess moisture.
4. Put the cauliflower back in the bowl and stir in the mozzarella cheese and egg.
5. Season with salt and black pepper and stir until well combined.
6. Spoon the mixture onto the baking sheet in two rounded

squares, as evenly as possible.

7. Bake for about 20 minutes until golden brown on the edges.

8. Mash the avocado with a pinch of salt and black pepper.

9. Spread the avocado onto the cauliflower toast and serve.

Nutrition Amount per serving

Calories 127 Total Fat 7g 9%

Saturated Fat 2.4g 12% Cholesterol 99mg 33%

Sodium 139mg 6%

Total Carbohydrate 9.1g 3% Dietary Fiber 4.8g 17% Total Sugars 3.4g

Protein 9.3g

APPETIZERS
AND
DESSERTS

Cheesy Radish

Serves: 5

Prep Time: 1 hour

Ingredients

- 16 oz. Monterey jack cheese, shredded

- 2 cups radish

- ½ cup heavy cream

- 1 teaspoon lemon juice

- Salt and white pepper, to taste

Directions

1. Preheat the oven to 3000F and lightly grease a baking sheet.
2. Heat heavy cream in a small saucepan and season with salt and white pepper.
3. Stir in Monterey jack cheese and lemon juice.
4. Place the radish on the baking sheet and top with the cheese mixture.
5. Bake for about 45 minutes and remove from the oven to serve hot.

Nutrition Amount per serving Calories 387

Total Fat 32g 41% Satu-

rated Fat 20.1g 100%

   Protein 22.8g

Cholesterol 97mg 32%

Sodium 509mg 22%

Total Carbohydrate 2.6g 1%

   Dietary Fiber 0.7g 3% Total

   Sugars 1.3g

Parmesan Garlic Oven Roasted Mushrooms

Serves: 6

Prep Time: 30 mins

Ingredients

- 3 tablespoons butter

- 12 oz. baby Bella mushrooms

- ¼ cup pork rinds, finely ground

- Pink Himalayan salt and black pepper, to taste

- ¼ cup parmesan cheese, grated

Directions

1. Preheat the oven to 4000F and lightly grease a baking sheet.
2. Heat butter in a large skillet over medium high heat and add mushrooms.
3. Sauté for about 3 minutes and dish out.
4. Mix together pork rinds, parmesan cheese, salt and black pepper in a bowl.
5. Put the mushrooms in this mixture and mix to coat well.
6. Place on the baking sheet and transfer to the oven.
7. Bake for about 15 minutes and dish out to immediately serve.

Nutrition Amount per serving

Calories 94

Total Fat 7.7g 10% Saturated Fat 4.7g 23% Cholesterol 22mg 7%

Sodium 228mg 10%

Total Carbohydrate 3g 1%

Dietary Fiber 0.9g 3% Total Sugars 1g

Protein 4.5g

Garlicky Green Beans Stir Fry

Serves: 4

Prep Time: 25 mins

Ingredients

- 2 tablespoons peanut oil

- 1 pound fresh green beans

- 2 tablespoons garlic, chopped

- Salt and red chili pepper, to taste

- ½ yellow onion, slivered

Directions

1. Heat peanut oil in a wok over high heat and add garlic and onions.
2. Sauté for about 4 minutes add beans, salt and red chili pepper.
3. Sauté for about 3 minutes and add a little water.
4. Cover with lid and cook on low heat for about 5 minutes.
5. Dish out into a bowl and serve hot.

Nutrition Amount per serving Calories 107

Total Fat 6.9g 9% Saturated Fat 1.2g 6%

Dietary Fiber 4.3g 15% Total Sugars 2.3g

Protein 2.5g
  Cholesterol 0mg 0%

Sodium 8mg 0%

Total Carbohydrate 10.9g 4%

Cheesy Low Carb

Creamed Spinach

Serves: 8

Prep Time: 25 mins

Ingredients

- 2 (10 oz) packages frozen chopped spinach, thawed
- 3 tablespoons butter
- 6 ounces cream cheese
- Onion powder, salt and black pepper
- ½ cup parmesan cheese, grated

Directions

Mix together 2 tablespoons of butter with cream cheese, parmesan cheese, salt and black pepper in a bowl.

1. Heat the rest of the butter on medium heat in a small pan and add onion powder.
2. Sauté for about 1 minute and add spinach.
3. Cover and cook on low heat for about 5 minutes.
4. Stir in the cheese mixture and cook for about 3 minutes.
5. Dish into a bowl and serve hot.

Nutrition Amount per serving

Calories 141

Total Fat 12.8g 16% Saturated Fat 8g 40%

Cholesterol 37mg 12%

Sodium 182mg 8%

Total Carbohydrate 3.5g 1% Dietary Fiber 1.6g 6%

Total Sugars 0.5g Protein 4.8g

PORK AND BEEF RECIPES

Cheesy Beef

Serves: 6

Prep Time: 40 mins

Ingredients

- 1 teaspoon garlic salt
- 2 pounds beef
- 1 cup cream cheese
- 1 cup mozzarella cheese, shredded
- 1 cup low carb Don Pablo's sauce

Directions

1. Season the meat with garlic salt and add to the instant pot.
2. Put the remaining ingredients in the pot and set the instant pot on low.
3. Cook for about 2 hours and dish out.

Nutrition Amount per serving

Calories 471

Total Fat 27.7g 36% Saturated Fat 14.6g 73%

Cholesterol 187mg 62%

Sodium 375mg 16%

Total Carbohydrate 2.9g 1% Dietary Fiber 0.1g 0%

Total Sugars 1.5g Protein 50.9g

Beef Quiche

Serves: 3

Prep Time: 30 mins

Ingredients

- ¼ cup grass fed beef, minced
- 2 slices bacon, cooked and crumbled
- ¼ cup goat cheddar cheese, shredded
- ¼ cup coconut milk
- 3 large pastured eggs

Directions

1. Preheat the oven to 3650F and grease 3 quiche molds.
2. Whisk together eggs and coconut milk in a large bowl.
3. Put beef in quiche molds and stir in the egg mixture.
4. Top with the crumbled bacon and cheddar cheese.
5. Transfer quiche molds to the oven and bake for about 20 minutes.
6. Remove from the oven and serve warm.

Nutrition Amount per serving

Calories 293

Total Fat 21.4g 27% Saturated Fat 10.4g 52% Cholesterol 232mg 77%

Sodium 436mg 19%

Total Carbohydrate 2.7g 1% Dietary Fiber 0.4g 2%

Total Sugars 1.1g Protein 21.8g

SEAFOOD RECIPES

Buttered Mahi Mahi Slices

Serves: 3

Prep Time: 30 mins

Ingredients

- ½ cup butter
- 1 pound Mahi Mahi, steamed and shredded
- ½ onion, chopped
- Salt and black pepper, to taste
- 1 mushroom, chopped

Directions

1. Preheat the oven to 3750F and grease a baking dish.
2. Mix together butter, onion, mushrooms, salt and black pepper in a bowl.
3. Make slices from the batter and place them on the baking dish.
4. Transfer to the oven and bake for about 20 minutes.
5. Remove from the oven and serve with a sauce.

Nutrition Amount per serving

Calories 445

Total Fat 32.1g 41% Saturated Fat 19.8g 99%

Cholesterol 224mg 75%

Sodium 390mg 17%

Total Carbohydrate 2g 1% Dietary Fiber 0.5g 2%

Total Sugars 0.9g

Protein 36.6g

Baked Mini Bell

Peppers

Serves: 4

Prep Time: 30 mins

Ingredients

- 1 oz. chorizo, air dried and thinly sliced

- 8 oz. mini bell peppers, sliced lengthwise

- 8 oz. cream cheese

- 1 cup cheddar cheese, shredded

- 1 tablespoon mild chipotle paste

Directions

1. Preheat the oven to 4000F and grease a large baking dish.

2. Mix together cream cheese, chipotle paste, bell peppers and chorizo in a small bowl.

3. Stir the mixture until smooth and transfer to the baking dish.

4. Top with cheddar cheese and place in the oven.

5. Bake for about 20 minutes until the cheese is golden brown and dish onto a platter.

Nutrition Amount per serving

Calories 364

Total Fat 31.9g 41% Saturated Fat 19.4g 97%

Cholesterol 98mg 33%

Sodium 491mg 21%

Total Carbohydrate 6g 2% Dietary Fiber 0.7g 2%

Total Sugars 2.9g

Protein 13.8g

CHICKEN AND POULTRY RECIPES

Keto Pesto Chicken Casserole

Serves: 3

Prep Time: 45 mins

Ingredients

- 1½ pounds boneless chicken thighs, cut into bite sized pieces
- Salt and black pepper, to taste
- 2 tablespoons butter
- 3 oz. green pesto
- 5 oz. feta cheese, diced

Directions

1. Preheat the oven to 400 F and grease a baking dish.
2. Season the chicken with salt and black pepper.
3. Heat butter in a skillet over medium heat and cook chicken for about 5 minutes on each side.
4. Dish out in the greased baking dish and add feta cheese and pesto.
5. Transfer the baking dish to the oven and bake for about 30 minutes.
6. Remove from the oven and serve hot.

Nutrition Amount per serving

Calories 438

Total Fat 30.4g 39% Saturated Fat 11g 55%

Cholesterol 190mg 63%

Sodium 587mg   26%

Total Carbohydrate 1.7g 1% Dietary Fiber 0g 0%

Total Sugars 1.5g Protein 39.3g

BREAKFAST
RECIPES

Chia Flaxseed Waffles

Total Time: 25 minutes Serves: 8

Ingredients:

- 2 cups ground golden flaxseed
- 2 tsp cinnamon
- 10 tsp ground chia seed
- 15 tbsp warm water
- 1/3 cup coconut oil, melted
- 1/2 cup water
- 1 tbsp baking powder
- 1 tsp sea salt

Directions:

1. Preheat the waffle iron.
2. In a small bowl, mix together ground chia seed and warm water.
3. In a large bowl, mix together ground flax seed, sea salt, and baking powder. Set aside.
4. Add melted coconut oil, chia seed mixture, and water into the blender and blend for 30 seconds.

5. Transfer coconut oil mixture into the flax seed mixture and mix well. Add cinnamon and stir well.
6. Scoop waffle mixture into the hot waffle iron and cook on each side for 3-5 minutes.
7. Serve and enjoy.

Nutritional Value (Amount per Serving):

Calories 240; Fat 20.6 g; Carbohydrates 12.9 g; Sugar 0 g; Protein 7 g; Cholesterol 0 mg;

Fresh Berries with Cream

Total Time: 10 minutes Serves: 1

Ingredients:

- 1/2 cup coconut cream

- 1 oz strawberries

- 1 oz raspberries

- 1/4 tsp vanilla extract

Directions:

1. Add all ingredients into the blender and blend until smooth.

2. Pour in serving bowl and top with fresh berries.

3. Serve and enjoy.

Nutritional Value (Amount per Serving): Calories 303; Fat 28.9 g; Carbohydrates 12 g; Sugar 6.8 g; Protein 3.3 g; Cholesterol 0 mg;

LUNCH
RECIPES

Asparagus Mash

Total Time: 20 minutes Serves: 2

Ingredients:

- 10 asparagus shoots, chopped
- 1 tsp lemon juice
- 2 tbsp fresh parsley
- 2 tbsp coconut cream
- 1 small onion, diced
- 1 tbsp coconut oil
- Pepper
- Salt

Directions:

1. Sauté onion in coconut oil until onion is softened.
2. Blanch chopped asparagus in hot water for 2 minutes and drain immediately.
3. Add sautéed onion, lemon juice, parsley, coconut cream, asparagus, pepper, and salt into the blender and blend until smooth.
4. Serve warm and enjoy.

Nutritional Value (Amount per Serving): Calories 125; Fat 10.6 g;
Carbohydrates 7.5
g; Sugar 3.6 g; Protein 2.6 g; Cholesterol 0 mg;

Creamy Squash Soup

Total Time: 35 minutes Serves: 8

Ingredients:

- 3 cups butternut squash, chopped
- 1 ½ cups unsweetened coconut milk
- 1 tbsp coconut oil
- 1 tsp dried onion flakes
- 1 tbsp curry powder
- 4 cups water
- 1 garlic clove
- 1 tsp kosher salt

Directions:

1. Add squash, coconut oil, onion flakes, curry powder, water, garlic, and salt into a large saucepan. Bring to boil over high heat.
2. Turn heat to medium and simmer for 20 minutes.
3. Puree the soup using a blender until smooth. Return soup to the saucepan and stir in coconut milk and cook for 2 minutes.
4. Stir well and serve hot.

Nutritional Value (Amount per Serving): Calories 146; Fat 12.6 g; Carbohydrates 9.4 g; Sugar 2.8 g; Protein 1.7 g; Cholesterol 0 mg;

BREAKFAST RECIPES

Bacon & Egg Fat Bomb

Healthy packed breakfast fat bombs that are guaranteed to satisfy you throughout the

morning.

Total Prep & Cooking Time: 50 minutes Level: Beginner

Makes: 3 Fat Bombs Protein: 2 grams

Net Carbs: 0.1 grams Fat: 13 grams

Sugar: 0 grams

Calories: 127

What you need:

- 1 large egg

- 12 cups of cold water, separated

- 1/4 tsp salt

- 3 tsp mayonnaise, sugar-free

- 1/8 cup butter

- 2 slices bacon

- 1/8 tsp pepper

Steps:

1. Fill a pot with 6 cups of the cold water and the eggs.
2. Set the timer for 7 minutes once the water starts to boil.
3. When the time has passed, drain the water and pour the remaining 6 cups of cold water on the eggs to halt the heating process.
4. Once cooled, peel the eggs and place in a dish with the butter, pepper, mayonnaise, and salt, whisking until combined.
5. Refrigerate for approximately half an hour.
6. Heat the bacon in a skillet until crispy and brown. Place on a plate with paper towels.
7. Crumble the bacon once cooled onto a small plate and remove the eggs from the fridge.
8. Scoop out small balls and cover entirely in the bacon bits, and serve immediately.

DINNER RECIPES

Almond Green Beans

Total Time: 20 minutes Serves: 4

Ingredients:

- 1 lb fresh green beans, trimmed
- 1/3 cup almonds, sliced
- 4 garlic cloves, sliced
- 2 tbsp olive oil
- 1 tbsp lemon juice
- ½ tsp sea salt

Directions:

1. Add green beans, salt, and lemon juice in a mixing bowl. Toss well and set aside.
2. Heat oil in a pan over medium heat.
3. Add sliced almonds and sauté until lightly browned.
4. Add garlic and sauté for 30 seconds.
5. Pour almond mixture over green beans and toss well.
6. Stir well and serve immediately.

Nutritional Value (Amount per Serving): Calories 146; Fat 11.2 g; Carbohydrates 10.9 g; Sugar 2 g; Protein 4 g; Cholesterol 0 mg;

DESSERT
RECIPES

Lemon Mousse

Total Time: 10 minutes Serves: 2

Ingredients:

- 14 oz coconut milk
- 12 drops liquid stevia
- 1/2 tsp lemon extract
- 1/4 tsp turmeric

Directions:

1. Place coconut milk can in the refrigerator for overnight. Scoop out thick cream into a mixing bowl.
2. Add remaining ingredients to the bowl and whip using a hand mixer until smooth.
3. Transfer mousse mixture to a zip-lock bag and pipe into small serving glasses. Place in refrigerator.
4. Serve chilled and enjoy.

Nutritional Value (Amount per Serving): Calories 444; Fat 45.7 g; Carbohydrates 10
g; Sugar 6 g; Protein 4.4 g; Cholesterol 0 mg;

LUNCH RECIPES

Egg Salad

Whip this egg salad up in no time and enjoy the fantastic boost in energy from this fat bomb.

Total Prep & Cooking Time: 15 minutes Level: Beginner

Makes: 2 Helpings

Protein: 6 grams Net Carbs: 1 gram Fat:

28 grams

Sugar: 1 gram

Calories: 260

What you need:

- 3 tbs mayonnaise, sugar-free
- 1/4 cup celery, chopped
- 2 large eggs, hardboiled and yolks separated.
- 1/2 tsp mustard
- 3 tbs red bell pepper, chopped
- 1/4 tsp salt
- 3 tbs broccoli, riced
- 1/4 tsp pepper
- 2 tbs mushroom, chopped
- 1/4 tsp paprika
- 4 cups cold water

Steps:

1. Fill a saucepan with the eggs and 2 cups of the cold water.

2. When the water begins to boil, set a timer for 7 minutes.

3. After the time has passed, drain the water and empty the remaining 2 cups of cold water over the eggs.

4. Once they can be handled, peel the eggs and remove the yolks. Chop the egg whites and leave to the side.

5. In a large dish, blend the mayonnaise, mustard, salt and egg yolks.

6. Combine the chopped celery, bell pepper, broccoli, and mushroom.

7. Finally, integrate the egg whites, pepper and paprika until combined fully.

UNUSUAL DELICIOUS MEAL RECIPES

Calamari Salad

This meal might look a little bit too unusual, but it will build your muscles after that powerful workout.

Total Prep & Cooking Time: 10 minutes Level: Beginner

Makes: 4 Helpings

Protein: 18 grams Net Carbs: 5 grams

Fat: 14 grams

Sugar: 0 grams

Calories: 214

What you need:

- 1/2 tsp lime juice
- 16 oz. calamari, sliced
- 1/4 tsp salt
- 2 tbs coconut oil
- 1/8 tsp pepper
- 8 oz. olives
- 1/2 tsp garlic powder
- 3 tsp coconut oil, separate
- 1/2 tsp lemon juice

Steps:

1. In a glass dish, blend the lemon and lime juice fully.

2. In a separate dish, whisk the 3 teaspoons of coconut oil, salt, garlic powder, and pepper until combined.

3. In a non-stick skillet, dissolve the 2 tablespoons of coconut oil with the olives. Heat the olives for about 90 seconds and remove to a serving plate.

4. Coat the calamari liberally in the seasonings.

5. Transfer the calamari to the hot oil and stir fry for approximately 2 minutes or until they become cloudy.

6. Remove to the serving plate with the olives.

7. Drizzle the juice dressing over the top of the plate and serve.

CAKE

Intermediate:

Lemon Cake

Serves: 10

Preparation time: 10 minutes Cooking time: 60 minutes

Ingredients:

- 4 eggs
- 2 tbsp lemon zest
- ½ cup fresh lemon juice
- ¼ cup erythritol
- 1 tbsp vanilla
- ½ cup butter softened
- 2 tsp baking powder
- ¼ cup coconut flour
- 2 cups almond flour

Directions:

1. Preheat the oven to 300 F/ 150 C.
2. Grease 9-inch loaf pan with butter and set aside.
3. In a large bowl, whisk all ingredients until a smooth batter is formed.
4. Pour batter into the loaf pan and bake in preheated oven for 60 minutes.

5. Slice and serve.

Per Serving: Net Carbs: 3.6g; Calories: 244; Total Fat: 22.3g; Saturated Fat: 7.3g Protein: 7.3g; Carbs: 6.3g; Fiber: 2.7g; Sugar: 1.5g; Fat 83% / Protein 12% / Carbs 5%

Fudgy Chocolate Cake

Serves: 12

Preparation time: 10 minutes Cooking time: 30 minutes

Ingredients:

- 6 eggs
- 1 ½ cup erythritol
- ½ cup almond flour
- oz butter, melted
- oz unsweetened chocolate, melted
- Pinch of salt

Directions:

1. Preheat the oven to 350 F/ 180 C.
2. Grease 8-inch spring-form cake pan with butter and set aside.
3. In a large bowl, beat eggs until foamy.
4. Add sweetener and stir well.
5. Add melted butter, chocolate, almond flour, and salt and stir until combined.
6. Pour batter in the prepared cake pan and bake in preheated oven for 30 minutes.
7. Remove cake from oven and allow to cool completely.
8. Slice and serve.

Per Serving: Net Carbs: 4g; Calories: 360; Total Fat: 37.6g; Saturated Fat: 21.6g

Protein: 7.2g; Carbs: 8.6g; Fiber: 4.6g; Sugar: 0.6g; Fat 90% / Protein 7% / Carbs 3%

KETO DESSERTS RECIPES

Cheese Chocolate Bars

Serves: 16

Preparation time: 10 minutes Cooking time: 10 minutes

Ingredients:

- 16 oz cream cheese, softened
- 14 oz unsweetened dark chocolate
- 1 tsp vanilla
- 12 drops liquid stevia

Directions:

1. Spray 8-inch square pan with cooking spray and set aside.

2. Melt chocolate in a saucepan over low heat.

3. Stir in sweetener and vanilla. Remove from heat and set aside.

4. Add cream cheese into the food processor and process until smooth.

5. Add melted chocolate mixture into the cream cheese and process until well combined.

6. Transfer cheese chocolate mixture into the prepared pan and spread evenly.

7. Place in refrigerator for 4 hours.

8. Slice and serve.

Per Serving: Net Carbs: 4.1g; Calories: 265; Total Fat: 23.1g; Saturated Fat: 14.5g

Protein: 5.5g; Carbs: 7.4g; Fiber: 3.3g; Sugar: 0.1g; Fat 82% / Protein 11% / Carbs 7%

COOKIES: BEGINNER

Simple Chocolate Cookies

Serves: 20

Preparation time: 5 minutes / Cooking time: 10 minutes

Ingredients:

- 3 tbsp ground chia
- 1 cup almond flour
- 2 tbsp chocolate protein powder
- 1 cup sunflower seed butter

Directions:

1. Preheat the oven to 350 F/ 180 C.
2. Spray a baking sheet with cooking spray and set aside.
3. In a large bowl, add all ingredients and mix until combined.
4. Make small balls from mixture and place on a prepared baking sheet.
5. Press lightly into a cookie shape.
6. Bake in for 10 minutes.
7. Allow to cool completely then serve.

Per Serving: Net Carbs: 4.2g; Calories: 111; Total Fat: 9.3g; Saturated Fat: 0.9g

Protein: 4g; Carbs: 5.2g; Fiber: 1g; Sugar: 0.2g; Fat 73% / Protein 13% / Carbs 14%

FROZEN DESSERT: BEGINNER

Raspberry Sorbet

Serves: 5

Preparation time: 10 minutes Cooking time: 10 minutes

Ingredients:

- 2 1/2 cups fresh raspberries
- 1 tbsp fresh lemon juice
- 1/3 cup erythritol
- 1/3 cup unsweetened coconut milk
- 1 tsp liquid stevia
- Pinch of sea salt

Directions:

1. Add all ingredients into the blender and blend until smooth.
2. Transfer blended mixture into the container and place in the refrigerator for 20 minutes.
3. After 20 minutes pour sorbet mixture into the ice cream maker and churn according to the machine instructions.
4. Pour into the air-tight container and place in the refrigerator for 1-2 hours.
5. Serve chilled and enjoy.

Per Serving: Net Carbs: 4g; Calories: 41; Total Fat: 1.9g; Saturated Fat: 0.7g

Protein: 1g; Carbs: 8g; Fiber: 4g; Sugar: 2.8g; Fat 45% / Protein 10% / Carbs 45%

BREAKFAST RECIPES

Broken Black Pepper Bread

Complete: 4 hr 45 min

Prep: 4 hr

Cook: 45 min

Yield: 1 portion bread

Nutritional Values:

Calories: 34, Total Fat: 5.1 g, Saturated Fat: 0.3 g, Carbs: 1.5 g, Sugars: 0.3 g, Protein: 1.3 g

Ingredients

- 2 cups in addition to 2 tablespoons milk
- 3 tablespoons unsalted spread
- 2 tablespoons sugar
- 1/2 teaspoons butcher's crush broke dark pepper
- One 1/4-ounce bundle dynamic dry yeast
- 5 cups generally useful flour
- 1 tablespoon fine salt
- Vegetable oil, as required

Direction

1. In a little pot, consolidate the milk, spread, sugar, and

pepper. Spot over medium-high warmth and achieve to 110 degrees F. Expel from the warmth and sprinkle the yeast over the outside of the milk. Put aside until frothy, around 10 minutes.

2. In the mean time, in an enormous bowl, whisk together the flour and salt.

3. Pour the milk and yeast blend into the bowl of flour and blend until a delicate, battered blend is shaped. Move the blend to a well-floured work surface and ply until a delicate versatile batter is framed, around 10 minutes. Move the mixture to a softly oiled bowl, spread with a kitchen towel, and spot in a warm spot, until puffed and multiplied in size, around 2 hours.

4. Spot a rack in the focal point of the broiler and preheat to 400 degrees F. Move the mixture to the work surface and, utilizing your hands, delicately straighten it into a 10-inch-long oval shape. Crease the batter into thirds longwise, covering the sides in the inside. Press down on the covering sides to seal and make a crease. Spot it crease side-down in a buttered 9 by 5- inch portion dish, spread with a kitchen towel, and come back to the hottest piece of the kitchen until the mixture has ascended around 1/2 crawls over the highest point of the container, around 1/2 to 2 hours.

5. Brush the highest point of the batter gently with warm water and, utilizing a sharp blade, make 1/4-inch-profound cut down the middle. Prepare until brilliant darker, around 30 minutes.

6. Expel the portion from the skillet and spot in the focal point of the rack. Keep heating until the portion sounds empty when riveted gently with your knuckles on the base and top, and a thermometer embedded in the inside peruses 200 degrees F., around 15 minutes.

7. Move the bread portion to a cooling rack and let cool for 2 hours before utilizing.

Tiramisu Cups

Preparation Time: 2 hours Servings:8

Nutritional Values:

Fat: 37 g.

Protein: 5 g.

Carbs: 5 g.

Ingredients:

For the Crust

- 1 cup Pecans, ground
- 1/3 cup Melted Butter
- 1 tbsp Unsweetened Cocoa Powder
- 2 tbsp Erythritol
- For the Filling
- 2 cups Mascarpone Cheese
- 1 shot Espresso
- ½ cup Erythritol
- 1 tsp Vanilla Extract
- 1 tbsp Gelatin
- 1 cup Boiling Water

Directions:

1. All ingredients should be combined for the crust in a bowl. Mix well. Pack the mixture into a silicon cupcake mold.

2. Combine gelatin and erythritol in a bowl. Stir in a cup of boiling water. Leave for 5 minutes.

3. Beat mascarpone cheese, espresso, and vanilla in a separate bowl until light and airy.

4. Gradually stir in the gelatin mixture into the whipped mascarpone.

5. Chill the mixture for 30 minutes.

6. Divide the mixture onto the cupcake mold and chill for an hour.

LUNCH RECIPES

Spicy Cloud Bread

Cooking time: 25-30 min Yield: 6 clouds

Nutrition facts: 52 calories per cloud: Carbs 2.8g, fats 3.4g, and proteins 3.1g.

Ingredients:

- 3 eggs
- 4 tbsp xylitol
- 2 tbsp cream cheese
- 2 tsp cinnamon, ground
- ½ tsp baking powder
- vanilla to taste

Steps:

1. Heat the oven to 175 C.
2. Prepare the baking sheet.
3. Beat the egg whites with baking powder for 2-3 min using a hand mixer until stiff peaks.
4. Mix yolks+cream cheese+vanilla+xylitol+cinnamon.
5. Combine whites with yolks softly.
6. Form 6 mounds and place the dough onto the baking sheet, greased. Make them flat.
7. Bake for 30 min until they are golden.

Soft Dinner Rolls

Cooking time: 20 min

Servings: 12 (2 rolls per serving)

Nutrition facts: 157 calories per serving: Carbs 4.5g, fats 13.2g, and 6.6g proteins.

Ingredients:

- 10 oz almond flour
- ¼ cup baking powder
- 1 cup cream cheese
- 3 cups mozzarella, shredded
- 4 eggs
- 1 tbsp butter

Steps:

1. Heat the oven to 190°C
2. Microwave mozzarella+cream cheese for a minute.
3. Mix all dry ingredients: almond flour+baking powder+eggs
4. Add cheeses to dry ingredients, mix well and put aside for 15 min.
5. Form 12 rolls and let them cool in the freezer for 7-10 min.
6. Melt the butter in the iron skillet.

7. Put the rolls next to each other and bake for 20 min in the skillet.
8. Enjoy

Notes:

So much quantity of baking powder will help the dough to rise well and not be flat.

SNACKS
RECIPES

Intermediate

Chaffle Fruit

Snacks

Preparation Time: 10 minutes

Cooking Time: 14 minutes

Servings: 2

Ingredients:

- 1 egg, beaten
- ½ cup finely grated cheddar cheese
- ½ cup Greek yogurt for topping
- 8 raspberries and blackberries for topping

Directions:

1. Preheat the waffle iron.
2. Mix the egg and cheddar cheese in a medium bowl.
3. Open the iron and add half of the mixture. Close and cook until crispy, 7 minutes.
4. Remove the chaffle onto a plate and make another with the remaining mixture.
5. Cut each chaffle into wedges and arrange on a plate.
6. Top each waffle with a tablespoon of yogurt and then two berries.
7. Serve afterward.

Nutrition:

Calories 207

Net Carbs 3.86g

Fats 15.29g

Protein 12.91g

Carbs 4.36g

Keto Belgian Sugar Chaffles

Preparation Time: 10 minutes

Cooking Time: 24 minutes

Servings: 4

Ingredients:

- 1 egg, beaten
- 2 tbsp swerve brown sugar
- ½ tbsp butter, melted
- 1 tsp vanilla extract
- 1 cup finely grated Parmesan cheese

Directions:

1. Preheat the waffle iron.
2. Mix all the ingredients in a medium bowl.
3. Open the iron and pour in a quarter of the mixture. Close and cook until crispy, 6 minutes.
4. Remove the chaffle onto a plate and make 3 more with the remaining ingredients.
5. Cut each chaffle into wedges, plate, allow cooling and serve.

Nutrition:

Calories 136

Fats 9.45g

Carbs 3.69g

Net Carbs 3.69g

Protein 8.5g

Lemon and Paprika Chaffles

Preparation Time: 10 minutes

Cooking Time: 28 minutes

Servings: 4

Ingredients:

- 1 egg, beaten
- 1 oz cream cheese, softened
- 1/3 cup finely grated mozzarella cheese
- 1 tbsp almond flour
- 1 tsp butter, melted
- 1 tsp maple (sugar-free) syrup
- ½ tsp sweet paprika
- ½ tsp lemon extract

Directions:

1. Preheat the waffle iron.
2. Mix all the ingredients in a medium bowl
3. Open the iron and pour in a quarter of the mixture. Close and cook until crispy, 7 minutes.
4. Remove the chaffle onto a plate and make 3 more with the remaining mixture.
5. Cut each chaffle into wedges, plate, allow cooling and serve.

<u>Nutrition:</u>

Calories 48

Fats 4.22g

Carbs 0.6g

Net Carbs 0.5g

Protein 2g

Herby Chaffle Snacks

Preparation Time: 10 minutes

Cooking Time: 28 minutes

Servings: 4

Ingredients:

- 1 egg, beaten
- ½ cup finely grated Monterey Jack cheese
- ¼ cup finely grated Parmesan cheese
- ½ tsp dried mixed herbs

Directions:

1. Preheat the waffle iron.
2. Mix all the ingredients in a medium bowl
3. Open the iron and pour in a quarter of the mixture. Close and cook until crispy, 7 minutes.
4. Remove the chaffle onto a plate and make 3 more with the rest of the ingredients.
5. Cut each chaffle into wedges and plate.
6. Allow cooling and serve.

Nutrition:

Calories 96

Fats 6.29g

Carbs 2.19g

Net Carbs 2.19g

Protein 7.42g

Breakfast Spinach

Ricotta Chaffles

Preparation Time: 10 minutes

Cooking Time: 28 minutes

Servings: 4

Ingredients:

- 4 oz frozen spinach, thawed, squeezed dry
- 1 cup ricotta cheese
- 2 eggs, beaten
- ½ tsp garlic powder
- ¼ cup finely grated Pecorino Romano cheese
- ½ cup finely grated mozzarella cheese
- Salt and freshly ground black pepper to taste

Directions:

1. Preheat the waffle iron.
2. In a medium bowl, mix all the ingredients.
3. Open the iron, lightly grease with cooking spray and spoon in a quarter of the mixture.
4. Close the iron and cook until brown and crispy, 7 minutes.
5. Remove the chaffle onto a plate and set aside.
6. Make three more chaffles with the remaining mixture.
7. Allow cooling and serve afterward.

Nutrition:

Calories 188

Net Carbs 4.06g

Fats 13.15g

Protein 12.79g

Carbs 5.06g

Pumpkin Spice

Chaffles

Preparation Time: 10 minutes

Cooking Time: 14 minutes

Servings: 2

Ingredients:

- 1 egg, beaten
- ½ tsp pumpkin pie spice
- ½ cup finely grated mozzarella cheese
- 1 tbsp sugar-free pumpkin puree

Directions:

1. Preheat the waffle iron.
2. In a medium bowl, mix all the ingredients.
3. Open the iron, pour in half of the batter, close, and cook until crispy, 6 to 7 minutes.
4. Remove the chaffle onto a plate and set aside.
5. Make another chaffle with the remaining batter.
6. Allow cooling and serve afterward.

Nutrition:

Calories 90

Fats 6.46g

Carbs 1.98g

Net Carbs 1.58g

Protein 5.94g

Mixed Berry-Vanilla Chaffles

Preparation Time: 10 minutes

Cooking Time: 28 minutes

Servings: 4

Ingredients:

- 1 egg, beaten
- ½ cup finely grated mozzarella cheese
- 1 tbsp cream cheese, softened
- 1 tbsp sugar-free maple syrup
- 2 strawberries, sliced
- 2 raspberries, slices
- ¼ tsp blackberry extract
- ¼ tsp vanilla extract
- ½ cup plain yogurt for serving

Directions:

1. Preheat the waffle iron.
2. In a medium bowl, mix all the ingredients except the yogurt.
3. Open the iron, lightly grease with cooking spray and pour in a quarter of the mixture.
4. Close the iron and cook until golden brown and crispy, 7 minutes.
5. Remove the chaffle onto a plate and set aside.

6. Make three more chaffles with the remaining mixture.

7. To Servings: top with the yogurt and enjoy.

Nutrition Facts per Serving:

Calories 78

Fats 5.29g

Carbs 3.02g

Net Carbs 2.72g

Protein 4.32g

Scrambled Egg
Stuffed Chaffles

Preparation Time: 15 minutes

Cooking Time: 28 minutes

Servings: 4

Ingredients:

For the chaffles:

- 1 cup finely grated cheddar cheese
- 2 eggs, beaten
- For the egg stuffing:
- 1 tbsp olive oil
- 1 small red bell pepper
- 4 large eggs
- 1 small green bell pepper
- Salt and freshly ground black pepper to taste
- 2 tbsp grated Parmesan cheese

Directions:

For the chaffles:

1. Preheat the waffle iron.
2. In a medium bowl, mix the cheddar cheese and egg.
3. Open the iron, pour in a quarter of the mixture, close, and cook until crispy, 6 to 7 minutes.
4. Plate and make three more chaffles using the remaining mixture.

For the egg stuffing:

1. Meanwhile, heat the olive oil in a medium skillet over medium heat on a stovetop.
2. In a medium bowl, beat the eggs with the bell peppers, salt, black pepper, and Parmesan cheese.
3. Pour the mixture into the skillet and scramble until set to your likeness, 2 minutes.
4. Between two chaffles, spoon half of the scrambled eggs and repeat with the second set of chaffles.
5. Serve afterward.

<u>Nutrition Facts per Serving:</u>

Calories 387

Fats 22.52g

Carbs 18.12g

Net Carbs 17.52g

Protein 27.76g

Ham and Cheddar

Chaffles

Preparation Time: 15 minutes

Cooking Time: 28 minutes

Servings: 4

Ingredients:

- 1 cup finely shredded parsnips, steamed

- 8 oz ham, diced

- 2 eggs, beaten

- 1 ½ cups finely grated cheddar cheese

- ½ tsp garlic powder

- 2 tbsp chopped fresh parsley leaves

- ¼ tsp smoked paprika

- ½ tsp dried thyme

- Salt and freshly ground black pepper to taste

Directions:

1. Preheat the waffle iron.

2. In a medium bowl, mix all the ingredients.

3. Open the iron, lightly grease with cooking spray and pour in a quarter of the mixture.

4. Close the iron and cook until crispy, 7 minutes.

5. Remove the chaffle onto a plate and set aside.

6. Make three more chaffles using the remaining mixture.

7. Serve afterward.

Nutrition Facts per Serving:

Calories 506

Fats 24.05g

Carbs 30.02g

Net Carbs 28.22g

Protein 42.74g

Savory Gruyere and Chives Chaffles

Preparation Time: 15 minutes

Cooking Time: 14 minutes

Servings: 2

Ingredients:

- 2 eggs, beaten
- 1 cup finely grated Gruyere cheese
- 2 tbsp finely grated cheddar cheese
- 1/8 tsp freshly ground black pepper
- 3 tbsp minced fresh chives + more for garnishing
- 2 sunshine fried eggs for topping

Directions:

1. Preheat the waffle iron.
2. In a medium bowl, mix the eggs, cheeses, black pepper, and chives.
3. Open the iron and pour in half of the mixture.
4. Close the iron and cook until brown and crispy, 7 minutes.
5. Remove the chaffle onto a plate and set aside.
6. Make another chaffle using the remaining mixture.
7. Top each chaffle with one fried egg each, garnish with the chives and serve.

Nutrition Facts per Serving:

Calories 712	Net Carbs 3.78g
Fats 41.32g	Protein 23.75g
Carbs 3.88g	

Chicken Quesadilla Chaffle

Preparation Time: 10 minutes

Cooking Time: 14 minutes

Servings: 2

Ingredients:

- 1 egg, beaten
- ¼ tsp taco seasoning
- 1/3 cup finely grated cheddar cheese
- 1/3 cup cooked chopped chicken

Directions:

1. Preheat the waffle iron.
2. In a medium bowl, mix the eggs, taco seasoning, and cheddar cheese. Add the chicken and combine well.
3. Open the iron, lightly grease with cooking spray and pour in half of the mixture.
4. Close the iron and cook until brown and crispy, 7 minutes.
5. Remove the chaffle onto a plate and set aside.
6. Make another chaffle using the remaining mixture.

7. Serve afterward.

Nutrition Facts per Serving:

Calories 314

Fats 20.64g

Carbs 5.71g

Net Carbs 5.71g

Protein 16.74g

Hot Chocolate

Breakfast Chaffle

Preparation Time: 10 minutes

Cooking Time: 14 minutes

Servings: 2

Ingredients:

- 1 egg, beaten
- 2 tbsp almond flour
- 1 tbsp unsweetened cocoa powder
- 2 tbsp cream cheese, softened
- ¼ cup finely grated Monterey Jack cheese
- 2 tbsp sugar-free maple syrup
- 1 tsp vanilla extract

Directions:

1. Preheat the waffle iron.
2. In a medium bowl, mix all the ingredients.
3. Open the iron, lightly grease with cooking spray and pour in half of the mixture.
4. Close the iron and cook until crispy, 7 minutes.
5. Remove the chaffle onto a plate and set aside.
6. Pour the remaining batter in the iron and make the second chaffle.
7. Allow cooling and serve afterward.

Nutrition Facts per Serving:

Calories 47

Fats 3.67g

Carbs 1.39g

Net Carbs 0.89g

Protein 2.29g

Blueberry Chaffles

Preparation Time: 15 minutes

Servings: 4

Ingredients:

- 2 eggs
- 1/2 cup blueberries
- 1/2 tsp baking powder
- 1/2 tsp vanilla
- 2 tsp Swerve
- 3 tbsp almond flour
- 1 cup mozzarella cheese, shredded

Directions:

1. Preheat your waffle maker.
2. In a medium bowl, mix eggs, vanilla, Swerve, almond flour, and cheese.
3. Add blueberries and stir well.
4. Spray waffle maker with cooking spray.
5. Pour 1/4 batter in the hot waffle maker and cook for 5-8 minutes or until golden brown. Repeat with the remaining batter.
6. Serve and enjoy.

Nutrition:

Calories 96

Fat 6.1 g

Carbohydrates 5.7 g

Sugar 2.2 g

Protein 6.1 g

Cholesterol 86 mg

Pecan Pumpkin

Chaffle

Preparation Time: 15 minutes

Servings: 2

Ingredients:

- 1 egg
- 2 tbsp pecans, toasted and chopped
- 2 tbsp almond flour
- 1 tsp erythritol
- 1/4 tsp pumpkin pie spice
- 1 tbsp pumpkin puree
- 1/2 cup mozzarella cheese, grated

Directions:

1. Preheat your waffle maker.
2. Beat egg in a small bowl.
3. Add remaining ingredients and mix well.
4. Spray waffle maker with cooking spray.
5. Pour half batter in the hot waffle maker and cook for 5 minutes or until golden brown. Repeat with the remaining batter.
6. Serve and enjoy.

Nutrition:

Calories 121	Sugar 3.3 g
Fat 9.7 g	Protein 6.7 g
Carbohydrates 5.7 g	Cholesterol 86 mg

Buns with cream cheese and cinnamon

Servings: 12

Cooking time: 40 minutes

Nutrients per one serving:

Calories: 81 | Fats: 11 g | Carbs: 3.5 g | Proteins: 10 g

Ingredients for the dough:

- ¾ cup almond flour
- 1 egg
- 2 tbsp cream cheese
- ½ tsp baking powder
- oz of mozzarella

Ingredients for filling:

- 2 tbsp cream cheese
- 3 tbsp stevia
- 2 tbsp water
- 2 tsp cinnamon

Cooking process:

1. The oven to be preheated to 180°C (356°F).
2. Grind the mozzarella. Add the cream cheese and heat in the microwave for 2 minutes. Add the flour, baking powder and egg to the cheese mass.

110

3. Mix well and knead the elastic dough. Divide into 8 round balls. Pull each part out into a long sausage and roll it out.

   4. Prepare the filling. In a bowl, mix 2 tablespoons stevia, cinnamon and water. Pour the filling on the dough. Form the tight sausage and cut into 10-12 buns.

   5. Put the buns on a baking sheet with parchment and bake in the oven for 25 minutes.

   6. Mix the cream cheese and 1 tbsp stevia. Lubricate hot buns with creamy dressing.

Sesame bread

Servings: 3

Cooking time: 20 minutes

Nutrients per one serving:

Calories: 82 | Fats: 12 g | Carbs: 1 g | Proteins: 7 g

Ingredients:

- 5 tbsp sesame flour
- 1 egg
- 1 tbsp butter
- ½ tsp baking powder
- A pinch of salt

Cooking process:

1. Mix the ingredients.
2. Melt the butter to room temperature.

Add butter and egg to the mass, mix well.

3. Pour the dough into a baking dish and bake in the oven at 180°C (356°F) for 15 minutes.

Chocolate Muffins

Nutritional Values:

Calories: 168.8, Total Fat: 13.2 g, Saturated Fat: 1.9 g, Carbs: 19.6 g, Sugars: 0.7 g, Protein:

1.1 g

Serves: 10 muffins

Wet ingredients:

- 2 oz medium Avocados, peeled and deseeded
- 4 Eggs
- 15-20 drops Stevia Drops
- 2 Tbsp Coconut Milk

Dry ingredients:

- 1 cup Almond Flour
- 1/3 cup Coconut Flour
- 1/2 cup Cocoa Powder
- 1 tsp Baking Soda
- 2 tsp Cream of Tartar
- 1/2 cup Erythritol
- 1 tsp Cinnamon
- Coconut Oil, for greasing

Directions:

1. Preheat your oven to 350F / 175C. Grease muffin cups with coconut oil and line your muffin tin.

2. Add the avocados to your food processor and pulse until smooth. Add the wet ingredients, pulse to combine until well incorporated.

3. Combine the dry ingredients and add to the food process and pulse to combine and pour the batter into your muffin tin.

4. Once crispy and baked for 20-25 minutes, remove from the oven and leave to cool before serving.

Pumpkin Cheesecake Chaffle

Preparation Time: 15 minutes

Servings: 2

Ingredients:

For chaffle:

- 1 egg
- 1/2 tsp vanilla
- 1/2 tsp baking powder, gluten-free
- 1/4 tsp pumpkin spice
- 1 tsp cream cheese, softened
- 2 tsp heavy cream
- 1 tbsp Swerve
- 1 tbsp almond flour
- 2 tsp pumpkin puree
- 1/2 cup mozzarella cheese, shredded

For filling:

- 1/4 tsp vanilla
- 1 tbsp Swerve
- 2 tbsp cream cheese

Directions:

1. Preheat your mini waffle maker.

2. In a small bowl, mix all chaffle ingredients.

3. Spray waffle maker with cooking spray.

4. Pour half batter in the hot waffle maker and cook for 3-5 minutes. Repeat with the remaining batter.

5. In a small bowl, combine all filling ingredients.

6. Spread filling mixture between two chaffles and place in the fridge for 10 minutes.

7. Serve and enjoy.

Nutrition:

Calories 107

Fat 7.2 g

Carbohydrates 5 g

Sugar 0.7 g

Protein 6.7 g

Cholesterol 93 mg

THE KETO LUNCH

Tuesday: Lunch:

Mason Jar Salad

So colorful and full of flavor. This salad is portable. Use any vegetable you have on hand.

Variation tip: try different kinds of protein, cheese or seeds.

Prep Time: 10 minutes Cook Time: None

Servings: 1

What's in it

- Cooked, diced chicken (4 ounces)
- Baby spinach (1/6 ounce)
- Cherry tomatoes (1/6 ounce)
- Bell pepper (1/6 ounce)
- Cucumber (1/6 ounce)
- Green onion (1/2 qty)
- Extra virgin olive oil (4 T)

How it's made

1. Chop vegetables.
2. Stuff spinach at the bottom of jar.
3. Layer the rest of the vegetables.
4. Keep olive oil in a separate container until ready to eat.

Net carbs: 4 grams Fat: 55 grams

Protein: 71 grams

Sugars: 1 gram

Wednesday: Lunch: The Smoked Salmon Special

This may be the easiest lunch special ever.

Flavorful, smoky, pink salmon poses on your

plate next to dark, green spinach as a feast for the eyes and the body.

Variation tip: serve with arugula or cabbage. Prep Time: 5 minutes

Cook Time: None Serves 2

What's in it

- Wild caught smoked salmon (.5 ounces)
- Mayonnaise (generous dollop)
- Baby spinach (large handful)
- Extra virgin olive oil (.5 T)
- Lime wedge (1 qty)
- Kosher salt (to taste)
- Fresh ground pepper (to taste)

How it's made

1. Place salmon (or any fatty fish like sardines or mackerel) and spinach on a plate.
2. Add a large spoonful of mayonnaise and the lime wedge.
3. Drizzle oil atop the baby spinach (or try arugula or cabbage shredded as if for slaw)
4. Sprinkle with a little salt and pepper. Net carbs: None

Fat: 109 gramsProtein: 105 grams Sugars: None

KETO AT DINNER

Monday: Dinner:

Beef short ribs in

a slow cooker

With a little prep, you will have a hot meal waiting for you at the end of a long day.

Variation tip: serve over diced cauliflower or with celery.

Prep Time: 15 minutes Cook Time: 4 hours

Servings: 4

What's in it

- Boneless short ribs or bone-in (2 pounds)
- Kosher salt (to taste)
- Fresh ground pepper (to taste)
- Extra virgin olive oil (2 T)
- Chopped white onion (1 qty)
- Garlic (3 cloves)
- Bone broth (1 cup)
- Coconut aminos (2 T)
- Tomato paste (2 T)
- Red wine (1.5 cups)

How it's made

1. In a large skillet over medium heat, add olive oil. Season meat with salt and pepper. Brown both sides.

2. Add broth and browned ribs to slow cooker

3. Put remaining ingredients into the skillet.

4. Bring to a boil and cook until onions are tender. About 5 minutes.

5. Pour over ribs.

6. Set to 4 to 6 hours on high or 8 to 10 hours on low.

Net carbs: 1 gram

Fat: 63 grams

Protein: 24 grams

Sugars: 1 gram

CPSIA information can be obtained
at www.ICGtesting.com
Printed in the USA
LVHW011022220221
679517LV00019B/1003